THE EXTENDED CARE UNIT IN A GENERAL HOSPITAL

A GUIDE TO PLANNING, ORGANIZATION, AND MANAGEMENT

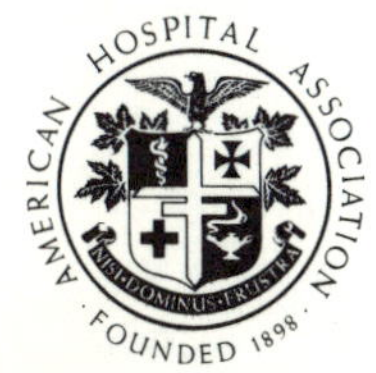

AMERICAN HOSPITAL ASSOCIATION · 840 NORTH LAKE SHORE DRIVE · CHICAGO, ILLINOIS · 60611

ISBN 0-87258-131-4
Library of Congress Catalog Card Number: 73-80342

840 North Lake Shore Drive
Chicago, Illinois 60611

Printed in the U.S.A.

M-60, Rev.
3M-6/73-3070

Text: 11 on 12 Baskerville

FOREWORD

The basic role of hospitals in long-term care is to provide, in partnership with other voluntary and governmental agencies, the necessary leadership for the development of a broad range of coordinated facilities and services for the chronically ill of all ages and for others requiring extended health services, in order to assure each patient adequate care in the right place, at the right time, and at a cost the nation, each community, and its citizens can afford.

Hospitals can and should exercise such leadership in a number of ways:

- They should promote vigorously the principles of areawide planning for convalescent, rehabilitative, and long-term care as an integral part of overall health care planning.
- They should recognize that their position—as institutions with organized medical staffs and a concentration of other professional personnel and specialized equipment—places upon them a major responsibility to extend the range and depth of their services. These services may include any or all of the following: rehabilitation programs; psychiatric services; extended care units; outpatient departments; day care, night care, and home care programs. The objective is a continuum of appropriate services centered about the patient.
- In communities where identified needs for health care of long-term patients are *not* being met because facilities and services are nonexistent, insufficient, or unacceptable, hospitals should consider the feasibility of providing such facilities and services (a long-term nursing care unit or a nursing home, for example) as an extension of their own programs.
- Where facilities for health care of long-term patients are sufficient and acceptable, hospitals should take the initiative in developing close working relationships with them.*

The objective is a system that assures continuity of care, coordination of services, and appropriate use of facilities and services.

*American Hospital Association. *Relationships among Health Care Facilities.* Chicago: AHA, 1965.

CONTENTS

"The hospital has established itself as the citadel of medical services in modern society. Enormous as the achievements of the past few decades have been, the changing needs of the public are demanding a changing hospital. . . .

"The concept of the hospital as a collection of the necessary physical facilities and personnel to provide medical care within its buildings or set of buildings is no longer viable in today's medical care system. The hospital now must be an organizational as much as a physical creature, an organized arrangement of all medical resources necessary to bring the individual, wherever located, into contact with the skills of his physician and other members of the health care team. It must serve as an arrangement by which our communities provide the organization, the people, the buildings, and the necessary materials and make available medical, nursing, and other professional care for the prevention, diagnosis, and treatment of disease, and eventually for the rehabilitation of the sick and injured, when these resources are beyond the capabilities of the individual patient or physician. At the center of this circle of medical resources must be the general hospital. This hub, the general hospital, cannot function independently of the other elements within the circle of organized hospital care activity, such as the outpatient departments, emergency departments, home care programs, and long-term care facilities. In addition, this wheel must be meshed with those preventive, curative, and rehabilitative health services that are outside the direct orbit of the hospital, such as visiting nurse services and school health programs."

— The Changing Hospital and the American Hospital Association. Chicago: American Hospital Association, 1965.

Chapter 1 INTRODUCTION

Most general hospitals, whether or not they operate an organized unit or a separate facility devoted to long-term patient care, do in fact have a considerable long-stay population. National Health Survey data show that during 1958-60 more than one-fourth of the total hospital days for patients discharged from short-term general hospitals represented stays exceeding one month. More recent surveys in individual hospitals have produced similar findings. The conclusion that general hospitals are in the business of serving long-term patients is inescapable.

Some hospitals are operating extended care units of various kinds. Others have units in the building or planning stage. Still others are just beginning to consider the feasibility of establishing such units. This guide was prepared to help all general hospitals benefit from the experience of pioneers in the development of these facilities; it highlights aspects of evaluation and planning that these pioneers consider important.

A study of long-term care facilities, discussed later in this chapter, provides data that should be of value to hospitals planning extended care programs. Conducted by the Medical Care Research Center, Washington University, St. Louis, it is a study of the characteristics of long-term care units in 143 general hospitals in 31 states.*

EXTENDED CARE UNIT—A WORKING DEFINITION

The term "extended care facility" was originally defined in Title 18 of the Social Security Amendments of 1965 (Public Law 89-97), which established Health Insurance for the Aged, or Medicare. The term refers to "an institution or a distinct part of an institution . . . which is primarily engaged in providing to inpatients (1) skilled nursing care and related services for patients who require medical or nursing care or (2) rehabilitation services for the rehabilitation of injured, disabled, or sick persons."†

This manual is concerned with one type of extended care facility: the extended care unit of the general hospital. The differentiation between such a unit and an acute care unit is based on (1) the phase of illness or disability of the patients served and (2) the scope and intensity of medical and nursing care provided. An extended care unit of a hospital can be defined as an inpatient nursing unit designed primarily for those patients whose condition is not acute but who still need an active medically oriented program of care that involves the regular and convenient availability of the resources of the hospital, such as its organized medical staff, its paramedical services, and its diagnostic and treatment facilities. These patients will usually require considerable rehabilitative nursing care and related medical and restorative services. The majority of them will not require this kind of care for a prolonged period of time and many of them will be ambulatory.

Among the patients who might appropriately be admitted to such an extended care unit are:

- A patient who has a *potentially recurrent disease,* such as bronchial asthma or congestive heart failure, and who needs careful observation in anticipation of a sudden attack.

*Rice, K. D. Organization of long-term care in general hospitals—a comparative study of patterns and practices in a national sample of general hospitals. Unpublished paper, Medical Care Research Center, Washington University, St. Louis, no date.

†The Social Security Amendments of 1972 (P.L. 92-603) provide for a single category of "skilled nursing facilities" that will be eligible to participate in both Medicare and Medical Assistance (Medicaid) for certain low-income persons. A "skilled nursing facility" will meet the prior definition of an extended care facility, as well as certain requirements of the Medicaid program.

- A patient who has a *potentially progressive disease,* such as diabetes mellitus, and who needs careful observation and supervision while learning to give himself necessary medications and to observe symptoms that must be watched for.

- A patient who has a *static handicap,* such as that resulting from an amputation or a stroke. The amputee will be adjusting to a new prosthesis; the stroke patient will be in the rehabilitation process.

- A patient whose *convalescence is prolonged* for one of a variety of reasons. For example: an older patient, or one in a poor nutritional state; a postcoronary patient whose tolerance, ability, and potential must be determined before discharge; or a patient who has had surgery that has made muscle retraining necessary, but who does not require intensive rehabilitation services.

- A patient with a *nonacute psychiatric condition.* Such a patient may not need psychiatric nursing care, but may need to be separated from a problem situation while receiving treatment.

The medical and nursing care needs of patients in these broad categories differ from those of acutely ill patients. Such appropriate candidates for admission to an extended care unit usually require less intensive nursing services and less frequent technical procedures than are provided in an acute care unit. Rapid changes in their conditions are less likely to occur, and the length of stay for the majority is relatively longer.

It should be noted that an extended care unit of a hospital is not the same as a minimal care or self-care unit. The latter is designed for persons who need little or no nursing care but who must be hospitalized for short periods while undergoing diagnostic studies or while learning to adjust to a medical regimen. Maximum self-care is, to be sure, one of the objectives of extended care, but most patients admitted to extended care units need practice and special training to achieve their full potential.

Extended care cannot, of course, be confined in a rigid or narrow definition. In the complete spectrum of interdependent services there is always an overlap of adjacent bands of care. The dimensions of the program of an extended care unit can be as flexible as the situation demands or allows, provided the program meets the needs of the patients admitted.

OVERALL NEED FOR A PLANNED PROGRAM

The development of organized programs for patients with illnesses or disabilities requiring nonacute care over an extended period of time has emerged as one of the major problems facing the voluntary health system. Census data, National Health Survey studies, special community studies, and individual hospital population studies combine to furnish abundant evidence that the needs for care of this increasingly large group of patients are not generally being met. These needs for care range widely in type and duration, although all patients in this group may properly be called long-term. The spectrum of facilities and services needed is equally broad; it includes general hospitals, special hospitals, and intensive rehabilitation centers; extended care facilities, including the extended care units of hospitals, nursing homes, personal care homes, and homes for the aged; and outpatient centers and home care programs.

Careful planning on an areawide basis is urgently needed to develop facilities in a coordinated pattern designed to bring into balance the diversity of health services for these patients (and for short-term patients as well). This pattern can be established only if the needs of all the people in the community are taken into account, and if individual institutions are willing to fit their own aspirations into a total plan for meeting these needs.

Several serious financial obstacles to the development of extended care facilities have been eased by a number of public and private approaches to the support of capital expansion, services, and the education and training of health manpower.

Financing for construction and modernization has been made available through the Hill-Burton grant and loan programs, administered by the Health Care Facilities Service in the U. S. Department of Health, Education, and Welfare.* A program of the Federal Housing Administration in the Department of Housing and Urban Development insures mortgages obtained by hospitals from private lenders.

*Continuation of support from this source was uncertain at the time of publication because it was not known whether the legislative authority for the Hill-Burton program would be extended beyond its expiration date of June 30, 1973.

Financing of extended care services is available through the Medicare program for the elderly and (as of July 1973) the disabled and through the Medicaid program for low-income individuals. Convalescent care for children may be covered under the Crippled Children's and Maternal and Child Health programs. Further, there is a growing trend to provide health care for retired members of the labor force and to develop coverage for long-term care under Blue Cross and private insurance plans.

Federal funds also are made available to hospitals, universities, and other organizations for the education and training of health care personnel.

A basic guide to federal support for health services and facilities is the *Catalog of Domestic Federal Assistance* published by the Office of Management and Budget in the Executive Office of the President.

RANGE OF PROGRAMS IN HOSPITALS

Long-term care units developed by general hospitals vary widely in character, but tend to be more numerous for patients who need an active medical program than for those whose primary need is personal care in a protective environment. Some hospitals administer more than one type of long-term care unit; for example, a rehabilitation unit and a chronic care unit, or an extended care unit and a nursing home facility. The range of services and the size of the units also vary greatly.

MEDICAL CARE RESEARCH CENTER STUDY

Some of the data provided by the study of the Medical Care Research Center of St. Louis will be referred to throughout the rest of this manual, and the implications of the findings will be used as the basis for various recommendations.* This was a study of a selected sample of long-term care facilities owned and maintained as units of voluntary general hospitals.

GROWTH IN LONG-TERM BEDS

One of the most important findings of the St. Louis study was that the overall growth of long-term beds in the 143 hospitals during the 10-year period between 1952 and 1962 exceeded the growth of

*Rice. *Op. cit.*

short-term beds. Almost three-quarters of the hospitals studied increased their long-term bed capacity, while less than one-half of the hospitals added short-term beds. (See table below.)

PATTERNS IN INCREASES, DECREASES, AND REALLOCATION OF BEDS IN 143 GENERAL HOSPITALS, 1952-62

Long-Term Pattern	Total Hospitals	Related Short-Term Pattern			
		No Change	Increase	Decrease	Reallocation
Total hospitals	143	38	68	12	25
No change	15	11	4	0	0
Increase	105	19	57	10	19
Decrease	10	6	3	1	0
Reallocation	13	2	4	1	6

Three types of activity were readily apparent: (1) the expansion of long-term facilities with corresponding expansion of short-term facilities; (2) the expansion of long-term facilities with reduction or no change in the number of short-term beds; and (3) the building of new short-term bed facilities, with conversion of the old ones for long-term beds. A fourth type of activity was more difficult to document: the practice of using long-term and short-term facilities interchangeably, depending upon patient demand. Many long-term units have been closed out periodically or permanently under pressure from medical staffs to use the beds for acutely ill patients.

Both the conversion of existing facilities to long-term use and the practice of using the same facilities interchangeably appear to have undesirable consequences. Although the physical plant does not necessarily determine the quality of care, the conversion of decrepit and obsolete facilities, or previously unusable space, for long-term use would suggest (and has a positive correlation with) low medical and administrative priorities for the extended care services. It also suggests marginal administrative opportunism; that is, an administration less interested in meeting patient needs than in keeping beds full, in meeting expenses, and in stabilizing services. The interchangeable use of facilities also frequently interferes with the development of the extended care program and the realization of its goals.

RELATIONSHIP BETWEEN ADMINISTRATIVE POLICIES AND QUALITY OF CARE

In the St. Louis study, an attempt was made to relate levels of care with certain kinds of administrative policies and procedures in use in the hospitals studied. Policies on admissions, and on a few related procedures immediately after admission, have been singled out for the purposes of this report. A consistent relationship was found to exist between what happens on admission and what happens later in treatment, transfer, and discharge.

The focus in this study was on care given, not solely on the physical plant, on the diagnostic or therapeutic equipment, or even on the trained personnel, though each is important. Levels of care are the result of what the hospital does with these resources rather than what the hospital's potential capability is.

In measuring the level of care in each hospital studied, the researchers considered three distinct groups of modalities. Scores were based on the availability and the extent of use of these modalities:

1. *Rehabilitative modalities,* including such services as physical therapy, occupational therapy, and recreational therapy.

2. *Maximal nursing care/medical modalities,* including services generally associated with an acute unit.

3. *Social modalities,* including minimal nursing services, with an emphasis on group living and dining, and recreational and diversional therapy.

Each extended care unit in the study was rated in each of the three areas and received a combination score. A unit that had indicated a specific type of service—that is, rehabilitation, chronic disease, or nursing home care—usually received scores that validated this claim. For example, nursing home units tended to receive high scores for the social modalities and lower scores for the maximal nursing care/medical modalities. In each case, it was assumed that more extensive use of the rehabilitative modalities, and of the professional nursing and medical modalities, was indicative of increased quality.

The broad groupings of units were based on this analysis:

Group A—Units with major emphasis on rehabilitative care and full utilization of hospital services:

1. Concern as to possible alternatives to admission to the extended care unit; emphasis on maximum services and reduction of unnecessary length of stay; and awareness of a need to develop and improve other services—both as alternatives

to admission and as acceptable outlets for discharge—were high in these units.

2. Evaluation procedures prior to admission included one or more of the following:

   a. Screening and evaluation in the acute section.

   b. Provision of any necessary intensive treatment in the acute section.

   c. Consultation with medical specialists.

   d. Examination by the medical director of the program.

   e. Clearance by a joint committee of representatives of the medical staff and the administration or by medical examination in the outpatient department.

3. Assignment of beds within the unit was based on the patient's need for access to medical attention, treatment areas, and nursing supervision.

Group B—Units with less emphasis on rehabilitative care and full utilization:

1. Evaluation procedures prior to admission included one or more of the following:

   a. Reliance on a medical examination submitted by the patient's physician.

   b. Clearance by a nonmedical administrator.

   c. Admission after an orientation conference between the hospital administrator and the patient's family.

2. Assignment of beds within the unit was based on sex, pay status, ambulatory status, and type and severity of impairment; concern seemed to be more for adjustment to the regimen than for access to needed services.

3. The unit's image was impaired by policies and procedures that gave credence to derogatory stereotypes of extended care units; such an image affected the attitudes of everyone involved as well as the effectiveness of the unit.

As a result of these observations, the following conclusions were drawn:

1. A nonmedical administrator should not be the single decision maker for an extended care unit.
2. The five types of evaluation procedures associated with units of Group A are correlated with a high degree of use of hospital facilities and tend to indicate high levels of care.

POTENTIAL SERVICE CAPABILITY AND ACTUAL SCOPE OF SERVICES

The survey also indicated that the good extended care programs usually get better, and the programs handicapped by lack of resources and services tend to get worse. Results of the study suggested that:

1. Hospitals that already have an adequate range of resources tend to improve the quality of extended care over time; such hospitals benefit from previous experience in the allocation and coordination of resources and personnel.
2. In hospitals without adequate service capabilities, extended care programs tend to become more narrow and inflexible over time; instead of improving quality, they reduce even further the range and quality of services available.

Lack of service capability, coupled with a desire to utilize marginal facilities at minimum operational cost, has produced long-term programs of poorer quality and inflexible structure in a large number of general hospitals.

Chapter 2 DETERMINING NEED FOR AND TYPE OF SERVICES

To meet the changing needs for health care facilities and services in a given community involves continuous planning. Every hospital has a planning responsibility. Accordingly, the hospital should have an active planning committee to examine its programs, to study the health needs of the surrounding area, and to develop short-term and long-range plans that are consistent with community needs and with the hospital's own special interest and capacity.

The hospital contemplating an extended care unit might wish to set up a committee for the special purpose of determining both the need for and the type of services. Such a committee would be, in effect, a subcommittee of the hospital's overall planning committee, working closely with that body and with the hospital's planning consultant if there is one. Its activities would necessarily take two directions: (1) review of the care needs of the hospital's own long-stay population and (2) evaluation of the community situation. Data collection in both areas could be going on concurrently.

REVIEW OF LONG-STAY PATIENTS IN HOSPITAL

Review of medical and administrative records will provide indications of needs for care. The participants in such a review should include representatives of the hospital administration and the medical and nursing staff, the medical record administrator, and the director of social service. Records of long-stay patients discharged during the past year or more, as well as those of patients presently under care whose stay is potentially long-term, should be analyzed. Pertinent information would include: the diagnostic category, prognosis, age and sex, the length of stay, the method and amount of payment, the source of referral, the location of patient's home (to define geographic area from which patients are drawn), the place to which the patient went on discharge and its suitability in terms of the individual's need for care, the degree of recovery and/or maintenance of gains as compared with the patient's potential, the number and type of readmissions. Later, follow-up studies on at least a representative sample might be required. Consultation from persons qualified to assist the committee in the design, conduct, and analysis of the review would be advisable.

In determining the potential use of an extended care unit, the amount and kind of nursing care that patients require is perhaps the primary consideration; this of course is related to the type and phase of their illness. However, it should also be borne in mind that patients must be selected on the basis of their total service needs. These needs include social as well as medical evaluation and treatment. If medical records are lacking in social data, it may be necessary to get additional information from other sources, at least for a representative group of patients in residence.

EVALUATION OF COMMUNITY NEEDS

The plans of one hospital are necessarily affected by the present and future plans of other hospitals and other health care institutions. All are affected by constantly changing conditions: scientific advances that may alter the disease spectrum or produce new treatment techniques; shifts in population; social changes; evolving patterns of housing, industrial growth, and transportation; increased means of financing care; availability of professional personnel; and many more.

Most large metropolitan areas are developing community health facilities planning agencies that involve both community leaders and staff people who presumably have community orientation. Ideally, such a planning body should be functioning in every area. It should be concerned with facilities and services for long-term health care as well as for acute care.

When an areawide planning group is already functioning, the hospital, of course, would be cooperating with it. Such a planning group would be the primary source of information concerning the need for extended health care in the community, the actual demand for services, and the availability of other resources—their type, quality, and utilization.

When a planning body does not exist, the hospital contemplating an extended care unit might wish to broaden the base of its exploratory subcommittee by adding representatives of the general medical community, public health, preventive medicine, and state health department, together with lay community leaders. The advantages of this approach are several: it guards against possible bias, ensures easier access to sources of necessary information, and, should the decision be to establish a unit, provides built-in support throughout the community.

Such a group—set up for the purpose of determining what kind of long-term care facility actually is indicated—would rarely undertake an exhaustive survey of overall community health needs. However, before considering any specific approach, the committee ought to have at least an estimate of how many people in the community are ill on a given day and where they are on that day. The following breakdown might be used:

- Total population.
- Number in short-term general hospitals.
- Number in nursing homes or related institutions (skilled nursing home, personal care home, residential home).
- Number in specialized institutions (rehabilitation center, children's hospital, other special hospitals).
- Number ill at home.
- Number getting care on an ambulatory basis (in physician's

office, in emergency and outpatient departments of hospitals, in clinics).

The question, of course, is whether these people are getting the care they need in the right place at the right time, or whether some who are presently in acute hospital units or in nursing homes, perhaps by default, would be better served in an extended care unit of the hospital. Even if a complete picture is unobtainable, any available information in these areas would be helpful in this exploratory stage.

SOURCES OF INFORMATION

Pertinent data are available from a number of sources. Under the Hill-Burton program, a designated state agency, most often the state department of health, has prepared plans for needed facilities and maintains information concerning acceptable beds in various categories of health facilities.*

Often the hospital facilities agency is also responsible for the licensing of such facilities. In any case, the licensing agency—whatever its auspices—can usually supply information about the quality of service provided by existing facilities and whether or not they are suitable for incorporation in the long-range planning pattern of the community.

Other possible sources of information and assistance are social, health, and welfare agencies; areawide planning agencies; local health departments; visiting nurse associations; the Red Cross; health and welfare councils; information and referral services; local and state medical societies; professors of preventive medicine and public health in teaching centers; hospital consultants; accepted accrediting bodies that evaluate various types of health facilities; metropolitan or state hospital associations; national health and hospital groups; third-party payers, including the Blue Cross and Blue Shield Plans; and the Federal Housing Administration (Department of Housing and Urban Development) and the Small Business Administration, which have records of applicants approved for loans.

Two joint committee reports of the American Hospital Association and the Public Health Service and a publication of the Hospital Review and Planning Council of Southern New York offer guidance

*See the annual *American Hospital Association Guide to the Health Care Field,* the list of State and Provincial Organizations and Agencies.

to local groups.* Individual hospital planning committees will find them equally valuable.

SUMMARY

With or without benefit of an areawide planning body or the kind of expanded committee suggested here, the hospital considering the need for undertaking an extended care program will have to evaluate the community situation in the perspective of the state plan and other sources, review the care needs of its own long-stay population, and then relate the two sets of findings. Even if the administrator is working with only a small, internal subcommittee, he can still get information from outside sources individually. For example, he could supplement a survey of the opinions of the hospital's medical staff with the views of other physicians in the local or county medical society, query health and welfare agencies and other sources, and consult third-party payers.

Hospitals should remember that each extended care bed frees an equivalent of at least two short-term beds. During the stay of a long-term patient transferred to an extended care bed, a series of patients with acute illness can be cared for and discharged in the short-term bed from which he was transferred. This is particularly important to hospitals considering the addition of short-term care facilities; the transfer of selected long-stay patients to an appropriate unit makes more short-term beds available and should result in more efficient utilization of all facilities.

---

*Joint Committee of the American Hospital Association and the Public Health Service on Areawide Planning of Hospitals and Related Health Facilities. *Areawide Planning for Hospitals and Related Health Facilities;* report. Washington, D.C.: U.S. Department of Health, Education, and Welfare, Public Health Service, Division of Hospital and Medical Facilities, 1961. (PHS Pub. No. 855)
Joint Committee of the American Hospital Association and the Public Health Service. *Areawide Planning of Facilities for Long-Term Treatment and Care;* report. Washington, D.C.: U.S. Government Printing Office, 1963. (PHS Pub. No. 930-B-1)
Hospital Review and Planning Council of Southern New York, Inc. *Guide and Suggested Procedures for Use by a Hospital Long-Range Planning and Development Committee.* New York: The Council, 1964.

Chapter 3

PLANNING THE EXTENDED CARE UNIT

Whenever possible, the planning committee should include persons who took part in determining extended care needs—particularly those persons who participated in the medical record review.

The planning group should include representatives of the medical staff, including both general practitioners and specialists from the various services likely to be involved in extended care—for example, medicine, orthopedics, surgery, physical medicine and rehabilitation, psychiatry, and neurology. The nursing staff, the administration, and the trustees should also be represented. Experience has shown, however, that high-level medical staff participation is the key to the success of an extended care program.

At appropriate times, when planning involves their special areas of competence or concern, other professionals should be called upon. They might include the director of social work, therapists in the rehabilitative services, residents (if the staff includes them), the director of admissions, the medical record administrator, the chief dietitian, and the chief engineer. It is suggested, however, that the basic planning committee be kept to a workable yet representative size.

PHILOSOPHY AND OBJECTIVES OF THE PROGRAM

Developing the philosophy and defining the goals and objectives of the unit should be the first job of the committee.

Objectives will not be identical for all hospitals; however, objectives are basic to subsequent decisions concerning program, staffing, location, design, and equipment. In a community with a full spectrum of services the role of the unit, along with its goals and objectives, may be definitely circumscribed; in another community with fewer resources, the hospital may have more latitude.

Because the concept of extended care is relatively new, it is especially important that the intent of the program be carefully considered and clearly stated at the outset. A written statement of the goals and objectives is particularly helpful.

As an example, the underlying philosophy of an extended care unit might be the belief that postacute patients need a total care program and will achieve their optimum potential more rapidly in a unit geared to their total needs—social, emotional, and spiritual, as well as medical; a unit in which the individual is not overlooked and in which the patient who is getting well receives just as much attention as the one who is more seriously ill; a unit in which personal independence is encouraged, in which restoration of function and training in self-help are emphasized; a unit in which the physical setting itself is beneficial to the patient because it has been designed to minimize hazards, to facilitate ease of movement, and to give patients more self-confidence during the training period; and one in which patients and their families receive assistance in making and carrying out plans for the future.

The broad objective of such a unit would be to provide post-acute care to selected patients who still need an active medically oriented hospital-based program as preparation for discharge to their own home, to a nursing home, or to a personal care facility.

The motivation for creating the unit will suggest more specific goals. They might include some or all of the following:

- To fill a gap in community resources.
- To improve utilization of medical and surgical beds by pro-

viding a more appropriate unit into which selected long-stay patients can be moved.

- To meet an anticipated increase in demand for extended care.
- To develop information about costs of extended care, per day and per patient.
- To furnish extended care at a lower cost than is possible for acute care.
- To stimulate interest of professional personnel in the problems of the chronically ill.
- To establish individual treatment goals for each patient.
- To ensure periodic evaluation of long-stay patients.
- To heighten interest in rehabilitative techniques and raise the level of rehabilitative care on all services.
- To reduce likelihood and number of readmissions.
- To prepare more patients for discharge to their own homes, thereby lessening the need for permanent institutionalization.
- To build a bridge between the hospital and other institutions providing long-term care facilities and services in the area, thereby making appropriate discharge arrangements easier to accomplish.
- To provide an appropriate place for readmitting patients who have been discharged to out-of-hospital programs such as home care or outpatient services.
- To train professional staff to work as a team in the active treatment of chronically ill and disabled patients.
- To offer educational experience with chronic illness to physicians, nurses, therapists, and other professional personnel in training.
- To demonstrate, and to educate the community in, the value of early rehabilitative care.

Long-term care is a dynamic process. It often requires reprogramming, restructuring, and refinancing; more often it requires reorientation of the medical staff. Failure to understand this can result in the loss of organizational control.

VARIATIONS IN EXTENDED CARE PROGRAMS OF HOSPITALS

It seems reasonable that hospitals planning to provide long-term care should give highest priority to the postacute needs of those chronically ill and disabled patients who can benefit most by the accessibility of the hospital's resources.

Two principles of planning for long-term care are especially pertinent here: (1) patient placement should be in accordance with need for service; (2) physical transfer of long-term patients should be minimized.* While facilities and services are likely to be used most effectively when long-term patients are placed according to their primary needs for service, frequent transfers of long-term patients occasioned by temporary changes in their needs for care are undesirable because of the emotional disturbances associated with dislocation. Thus, it is desirable to provide in the unit a range of services sufficiently broad to minimize physical transfers, which thus would be necessitated only by pronounced changes, likely to persist for an extended period, in the patient's needs for care.

Thus, extended care units in general hospitals are often "mixed," in that they provide several kinds of services; this can create problems. However, if a mixed service is needed, the hospital should at least be fully aware of what is mixing and should establish a system of priorities to maintain a balance. Sometimes actual experience modifies initial objectives, with the result that a broader range or mixing of services is provided. Though this may be desirable, within limits, it can subvert the original purpose of the unit to such an extent that a sound program of long-term care cannot be carried out. For example, if the unit admits patients for convalescent or diagnostic stays of only a few days as well as the chronically ill, it may end up being little different from the acute care units of the hospital. On the other hand, if the unit admits or retains patients who need only custodial care, it can rapidly become only a custodial unit.

Findings in the St. Louis study,† among others, substantiate the risks involved when the extended care unit accepts patients who do not require its special services or retains patients after they have ceased to benefit from these services. Therefore, it is particularly important that admission and discharge policies be carefully considered.

**Areawide Planning of Facilities for Long-Term Treatment and Care,* pp. 27, 28.
†Rice. *Op. cit.*

DETERMINATION OF ADMISSION AND DISCHARGE POLICIES

Admission and discharge policies should be concretely formulated consistent with the unit's objectives and reinforced by a mechanism for ensuring that they are carried out.

ADMISSION

Types of patients cared for. In making decisions concerning the types of patients to be cared for in the unit, answers to the following questions are particularly pertinent:

- Will rehabilitation be particularly emphasized, and will patients for the most part be rehabilitation candidates?
- If the hospital has a rehabilitation unit, what considerations will guide placement in that unit as opposed to the extended care unit?
- Will admissions be limited to medical patients or will others—such as postsurgical and orthopedic patients—be accepted?
- Will certain patients be ineligible? Those with chronic communicable conditions? Those with psychiatric conditions such as acute anxiety, psychotic reactions, alcoholism, drug addiction? Those requiring oxygen service, surgical intervention, frequent blood transfusions, intravenous feeding, therapeutic diets? Those with terminal conditions?

The spectrum of services available in the community will have an effect on these policy decisions, as will the amount of intensive nursing care required by the patient.

Age range of patients. Such a decision is also important to the development of the program. To avoid concentration on the aged, it is recommended that patients be accepted from a wide range of age groups.

Source of admissions. In planning the unit, decisions will have to be made in answer to the following questions:

- Will direct admission to the unit, as to other departments, be permitted?
- Will transfers from another hospital, a nursing home, or other care facilities in the community be accepted? Which ones will have priority?
- Will nonstaff physicians be permitted to admit patients?

Physician's responsibility. Policy decisions in this area would involve requirements concerning the complete history and other special information for referred patients; the advisability of specifying minimum frequency of visits; the determination of responsibility for developing individual care plans, for periodic evaluation of patient's progress, and for the handling of emergency situations; and so on.

DISCHARGE

Well-defined discharge policies are just as important as well-defined admission policies. Factors to be considered include the following:

Maximum length of stay. It is desirable to stipulate the period of time after which discharge to the patient's home or to another facility is expected unless there is medical justification for the extension of the patient's stay. Such a stipulation, however, will be ineffective without provision of a specific and widely understood mechanism to implement it.

Continuing care. Provisions for continuing care, when it is needed, should be made a part of the discharge procedure. The importance of early planning for discharge or transfer from both the acute units and the extended care unit cannot be overemphasized. Formal agreements expedite transfers to other facilities and services; they are strongly recommended.

When the committee has thought through the objectives of the unit, the types of patients it will serve, and some of the rules that will apply, the hospital might consider evaluating these policies and procedures in relation to its own patient population. If problems are encountered, some rethinking should be done. At this point it might also be helpful to visit other hospitals where similar programs are in operation.

PHYSICAL RELATIONSHIP TO HOSPITAL

It is generally agreed that the extended care unit should be contiguous to the main hospital, primarily to provide accessibility to medical staff and to the hospital's service areas. All evidence collected in the St. Louis study* points to the fact that physically separated facilities, or facilities that do not provide easy access to

*Rice. *Op. cit.*

other hospital areas, are not conducive to a high quality of extended care services. For example, if the physical therapy department is very far from the extended care unit, it is difficult to find time and personnel to transport the patients to the physical therapy department. Such hindrances as stairs, open sidewalks, and streets greatly hamper the movement of patients and personnel.

The study also revealed, however, that if the extended care facility is not physically distinct from acute medical and surgical areas, multiple forms of organizational stress are likely to occur. The presence of chronic extended care patients often has a depressing effect on short-term patients and their families.

The optimum arrangement would seem to be a nursing unit that is separate but that remains an integral part of the hospital, not an isolated outpost. The advantages to such an arrangement are several:

1. *Identification as a hospital nursing unit.* Integration minimizes the danger of the extended care unit being considered a nursing home, an old-folks home, a geriatric unit, or something similar, connoting an age category of the patients.
2. *Convenience for medical staff visitations.* The tendency toward subtle disengagement is lessened if the unit is right at hand. If physicians are to become acquainted with the unit's policies and operation, take an interest in its success, and use it, it must be easily accessible during their daily hospital rounds.
3. *Improved service to the patient.* Proximity facilitates access to ancillary services such as x-ray, laboratory, and pharmacy; closer and more frequent contact with rehabilitation personnel; availability of other specialized personnel such as social workers, dietitians, medical record administrators; smooth transfer of patients from the acute sections to the unit, or the reverse, as their needs change.
4. *Training of personnel.* The attached unit offers opportunities for training all types of personnel in the care and rehabilitation of longer-term patients.
5. *Economy of operation.* Economies include utilization of basic facilities and services such as kitchens, laundry, heating, lighting, maintenance, joint purchasing, and a single administration.

One disadvantage cited by some people is that the physically attached unit tends to be more hospital-like in atmosphere than the separate facility. However, careful attention to design can provide an environment satisfying and pleasant to the extended care patient.

SIZE

Considerations in determining the size of the extended care unit include both the number of beds, within an economically feasible range, and the percentage of total hospital beds.

NUMBER OF BEDS

Optimum size of the nursing unit will depend on many factors including condition of patients selected for treatment; however, a range of 30 to 60 beds is generally considered proper in extended care. The unit should be large enough to be economical and functional. Its size should justify a sufficient number of full-time professional personnel during the busy periods of the day to characterize it as a separate nursing unit; and during evening and night shifts it should be able to utilize one or two staff people.

A 20-20 or a 30-30 arrangement, with the nurses' station located between the two groups of beds, facilitates evening and night supervision by a reduced staff.

Where existing facilities are being adapted or remodeled, restrictions on size may be automatic. If the physical limitations are too great, the feasibility of using the available space may have to be reconsidered; incorporation of the unit as part of another unit is not recommended.

PERCENTAGE OF TOTAL BEDS

The proportion of long-term beds to short-term beds is an equally important consideration. There are dangers in allowing the former to exceed the latter. A general hospital with a high proportion of long-term beds (40 per cent or more) can all too easily become known as a geriatric or chronic hospital. Medical, administrative, and social stereotypes form quickly about this type of specialization. Selective referral and admission of nothing but extended care patients may develop before management is fully aware of the trend. Once such a trend starts, it is extremely difficult to reverse it;

and the specific hospital is no longer considered a general medical facility. This problem, of course, is most serious for the smaller hospital.

The appropriate range of the percentage of extended care beds in a general hospital is estimated to be from 10 to 35 per cent. With this as a guide, the number of extended care beds should be governed both by whether the number comes within the appropriate range and by whether it is economically feasible.

REQUIRED SERVICES

Rehabilitation nursing under proper medical supervision is essential for any extended care unit. Other basic service requirements will be determined to a large extent by the objectives of the unit, the kinds of patients to be treated, and the phase of their illness. Access to social service and the rehabilitative services such as physical and occupational therapy is also essential in most cases.

As was noted in the St. Louis study,* good extended care programs—those that provide an adequate range of services—tend to get better, and programs handicapped by the lack of resources and services tend to become less effective. To guard against the latter possibility, hospitals should focus simultaneously on (1) accelerating the use of diagnostic and clinical services and (2) developing basic rehabilitative services either independently or through cooperative arrangements with other health care facilities. It would appear that one important measure of quality of extended care is the amount of time that elapses between a patient's readiness for rehabilitation services and his receiving them.

Today, many general hospitals are not equipped to provide a full range of extended care services. There is a real question whether these smaller hospitals should even consider the operation of an extended care program as such. Unless services requisite to the full range of the patient needs can be developed prior to or simultaneously with the opening of the unit, the hospital might well consider alternatives to establishing an extended care program. For example, it might be more expedient to develop various affiliations with larger institutions in the area. In transferring patients, however, the hospital should take adequate steps to ensure that the restorative potential of each patient is evaluated by capable professional per-

*Rice. *Op. cit.*

sonnel and that the patient's potential for restoration of function is not impaired by delay of transfer.

DESIGN, CONSTRUCTION, EQUIPMENT

The design and construction of the unit and the equipment to be used in it are affected by the special needs of extended care patients. A discussion of the additions to and modifications of facilities required for such patients is included here; facilities that are the same as for any other unit—nurses' stations and linen storage areas, for example—are not discussed.

GENERAL CONSIDERATIONS

All areas—patient rooms, treatment areas, corridors, doorways, elevators, lounge and dining areas—must be spacious enough to accommodate wheelchairs, walkers, and stretchers; the turning radius of a wheelchair becomes a module of design.

Mechanical fixtures and controls should be placed within easy reach of a patient in a wheelchair. This includes silent light switches, nurse call buttons, lavatory handles, sinks, soap and towel dispensers, shelves, mirrors, clothing storage space and hangers, drinking fountains, telephones, elevator call buttons, and self-service controls.

Entrance doors should be automatically operated; other doors should open with a minimum of resistance. Where possible, thresholds should be eliminated and gradual ramps should be substituted for stairs if differences in elevation cannot be avoided. Handrails are helpful in certain areas, though their use should be closely supervised. If long corridors are unavoidable, resting spots should be provided.

The use of carpeting in an extended care unit warrants particular consideration. Not only is it easy to maintain; it reduces noise and make the unit more homelike and attractive. Considerations in carpet selection should include characteristics relating to smoke and toxic gases, durability, and ease of movement of wheels and rollers. It should also be pointed out that in many states the licensing agency requires that samples of carpeting be submitted and tested by the agency; in some states use of carpeting in health care facilities is prohibited.

A ground floor location—accessible to the outdoors—is preferable for an extended care unit. However, if the only way the building can expand is upward, a roof garden might be considered; natural light and fresh air are valuable assets.

Air conditioning should be considered. In some climates it might not be necessary, though the public may demand it. The therapeutic benefits of air conditioning should also be studied with respect to appropriate levels of humidity. If air conditioning is to be installed at a later date, the original structure should be built to accommodate a central system or small units, as desired. If central air conditioning is to be installed, an individual temperature control mechanism for each room is advisable.

SPECIFIC CONSIDERATIONS

Patient rooms. The room requirements of extended care patients are different from those of acute patients in several respects.

A high percentage of private rooms in this unit is advocated by some on the grounds that longer-stay patients need intervals of complete privacy; they have ample opportunity for socializing in the dining room-lounge. Another advantage of the private room is reported to be greater flexibility in the placement of patients. Others, however, believe that the need for mutual encouragement and camaraderie is particularly important and can be better met in double rooms and wards. Patient preferences will vary according to type and phase of illness, temperament, sociological background, psychological reaction to illness, and the like. Since charges for private room occupancy are usually higher than charges for other accommodations, ability to pay also becomes a consideration.

The desirable ratio of private rooms to double rooms and wards will depend on many factors, including established patterns of use of the acute care facilities and reimbursement policies of third-party payers. Experience shows, however, that an all-private room 400-bed general acute hospital is roughly equivalent to a 450-bed multiple-and-private room hospital; for a variety of reasons, 10 to 20 per cent of the beds in two-bed rooms are not being used. The situation in an extended care unit would be similar, though the percentage of unused beds might be somewhat lower.

Room furnishings and equipment. Several different types of beds should be considered for an extended care unit; these range from the all-electric completely adjustable bed to the manually adjustable high-low bed to the standard or improved dormitory type. Needs will vary with the type of patients to be cared for.

Showers, tubs, toilets, and lavatories in patient rooms must be specially designed to accommodate wheelchair patients and to facilitate self-care. Grab bars and other such features are needed. Suitable wardrobes or adequate closet and drawer space are particularly important to long-stay patients.

If policies of the unit exclude care of patients requiring oxygen and suction on a routine basis, such special equipment should not be installed. Provision of emergency equipment as a standby is perhaps more appropriate.

Since many extended care patients are likely to be ambulatory and to have a fair number of visitors, an ample amount of comfortable and functional furniture is important. Suggested is at least one high-back chair for the patient to lounge and relax in when he is up. An accompanying ottoman would not only increase his comfort but could also double as a seating piece during visiting hours. If possible, several side chairs should be provided. Curtains and pictures add attractive touches; the tasteful use of color creates a pleasant effect.

Treatment areas. Detailed information on such specialized services as physical therapy, occupational therapy, and social work can be found in other American Hospital Association manuals devoted to those subjects. Central rehabilitation services would not be duplicated, of course, but space and equipment for occupational therapy might be provided to permit a supplementary program.

Central bathing facilities. Because of their efficiency of use, a maximum ratio of showers to tubs is recommended; experience has shown the particular advantage of showers that can be entered by patients in wheelchairs. Individual units, with waist-high dividers to keep the attendant dry while he assists the bather, are recommended, as are gooseneck shower head attachments that can be adjusted for standing or sitting. Minimum Hill-Burton requirements for various types of long-term facilities should, of course, be met; they should be exceeded wherever indicated.

Lounge-dining areas. Properly designed and equipped, these areas can easily be converted from one use to the other. Space set aside on each floor should be adequate to accommodate a majority of the patients. It is wise to select multipurpose furniture such as tables that can be extended to seat six or eight at mealtime, then contracted to card-table size; their design should also permit use by wheelchair patients. To achieve a homelike atmosphere, a mixture of functional dining furniture and comfortable lounge furniture is advisable.

Storage space. Because of the type of patient served and the length of the patients' stay, it is necessary to plan storage space for wheelchairs, luggage, and so forth.

Activities-of-daily-living area. A special area equipped for teaching all of the activities of daily living is desirable in some facilities. Much of the equipment used in such an area can be accommodated in the nursing care areas.

Patient library. This is an optional facility, much appreciated by many patients. It also provides another area that is separate from the nursing unit—often a welcome relief from the confinement there.

Chapel. Many hospitals provide a chapel or a meditation room for the patients. If it is of adequate size and conveniently located, it certainly should be used by extended care patients. However, if such a room is not available, it should be considered.

SOURCES OF INFORMATION

Information on construction and design of extended care units is available from a number of sources, and it is wise to consult several of them. (See General References at the end of this manual.) State health departments and other health agencies can provide useful information, particularly since requirements differ for the various types of units; requirements also differ from state to state. Information obtained from visits to other facilities having similar objectives can be helpful.

A good architect is indispensable, of course. However, it is the responsibility of the administration's planning committee to furnish the architect with detailed written information concerning the function, purpose, and requirements of each area of the unit.

ESTIMATING NURSING STAFF NEEDS

All staffing estimates for an extended care unit must be based upon the purposes of the unit and the medical care goals established for the patients who will occupy the unit. Since nursing care is the primary focus in most extended care units, the staffing of this department is considered first.

The medical and nursing staff of the hospital should analyze the medical care needs of prospective patients in terms of the projected goals—the degree of assistance necessary to maintain personal hygiene, the kinds and complexities of therapeutic regimens indicated, the extent to which teaching self-help is anticipated, and so on. On the basis of this analysis, decisions can be made as to the kinds and number of personnel required and the kind of preparation they should have—registered nurses, licensed practical nurses, nursing aides, and ward clerks.

Professional nursing supervision should be available around the clock. The number of registered nurses required, in addition to a specially qualified supervisor who has overall nursing responsibility for the unit, will depend upon the nursing needs of patients and the degree of supervision necessary for supportive personnel. Nursing care on an extended care unit is usually less technically complex than on an acute medical or surgical unit, and a lower ratio of registered nurses to licensed practical nurses and well-trained nursing aides is often possible.

There are differing points of view, however, concerning ratios of registered professional nurses to other nursing personnel. Experience reported by the Loeb Center for Nursing and Rehabilitation at Montefiore Hospital in New York City suggests that employment of only registered professional nurses produces a more effective nursing care program at less cost.* Presumably this is because professional nurses can devote all of their time to nursing; time that would otherwise be given to on-the-job training and close supervision of other personnel is obviated. The more productive man-hours of nursing time thus result in a lessening of the need for personnel.

Because patients' need for care during night hours is usually limited, reduced staffing for that period may also be possible. Rehabilitative nursing and the promotion of self-care are time consuming; they require special skills. In many ways the demands on staff in an extended care unit are different from those in an acute care unit, but it does not follow that they necessarily are less.

According to statistics collected by Hospital Administrative Services of the American Hospital Association in 1964, an average of 3.3 available man-hours of nursing personnel per bed was reported for extended care units in one state. Of this, 20 per cent was professional nursing time and 80 per cent was nonprofessional. It must be emphasized that these statistics are not equated with the quality of nursing care and should not be considered a standard.

*Hall, L. E. A center for nursing. *Nurs. Outlook* 11:805, Nov. 1963.

They are reported here only to give some indication of minimums to be considered in estimating staffing requirements.

ESTIMATING COSTS AND FINANCING

CAPITAL COSTS AND FINANCING

Costs of constructing and equipping an extended care unit vary greatly in relation to the services to be provided in the unit and in relation to the adequacy of the hospital's supporting services.

If, for example, the dietary, laundry, x-ray, and clinical laboratory services of the hospital can serve the extended care unit without physical expansion, the per-bed cost of construction for this unit will be lower than the per-bed cost of a medical-surgical unit of comparable size.

Other factors that can lower capital costs include the probable omission of piped-in oxygen, built-in suction apparatus, physiological monitoring equipment, and electronic bedside consoles. Soundproofing is also considered by some to be a less important feature in extended care units than in general medical-surgical units.

The availability of capital financing must be assured before plans can proceed. Potential sources of funds include the usual ones —tax revenues, loans, contributions from charitable organizations and foundations or from individuals through fund-raising campaigns and bequests. Support for construction and modernization of extended care facilities under the Hill-Burton program is obtained through application to the designated state agency. A number of states have developed programs of direct grant assistance to qualified sponsors of needed facilities. Mortgage loan insurance is provided to both not-for-profit and for-profit applicants through the Federal Housing Administration in the Department of Housing and Urban Development.

OPERATING COSTS AND FINANCING

Adequate financial support for maintaining and operating an extended care facility is vital. With only one or two exceptions, financial support has the greatest influence on the quality and utilization of the extended care unit.

Operating costs—both direct and indirect—must be estimated as accurately as possible before charges for care can be established.

These costs include salaries, supplies, and miscellaneous expenses for services directly provided by the unit—primarily nursing service —plus that portion of the cost of jointly shared services that is attributable to the unit and that must be allocated to its operating costs. Examples of the jointly shared services would be special services such as dietary service, rehabilitation, social service, pharmacy, medical records, and central supply room, as well as laundry, housekeeping, plant maintenance, and so on.

Some hospitals report a markedly lower use of laundry services by the extended care units, while others report the same or higher use in comparison with other nursing units. This variation can probably be attributed to the kinds of patients accepted. For example, if there are considerable numbers of incontinent patients, laundry use will be higher. The additional demands for food service, on the other hand, are approximately the same as they would be for any other nursing unit.

Nonoperating expense consists chiefly of depreciation and financing costs; such items must be included in overall cost estimates.

General experience with extended care units to date indicates that costs are roughly one-half to two-thirds of the average per diem cost in an acute unit, depending, of course, upon the size of the extended care unit and the range of services. However, this differential should not be taken for granted. Cost estimates should be based on a thorough analysis, and the allocation of costs should be realistically considered. While it may be feasible to begin with a minimal operation in terms of size and then expand the unit if and when demand increases, the basic services required by the kinds of patients to be accepted should be available at the outset and the cost for these basic services must be considered in the planning.

ESTABLISHING CHARGES

The administration must weigh many considerations before the method of charging and the rate of charges are decided. The decision must be made whether charges for the unit will be made on the basis of an all-inclusive or a semi-inclusive rate, or whether separate charges will be made for various individual services, such as increased nursing service necessitated by incontinence, special diets, and so on—a customary practice in nursing homes.

How important is it that the charging system for acute services and that for services on the extended care unit be the same? Typically, the hospital makes a daily service charge and makes a separate charge for ancillary services only. It might be difficult, then, to use a different system of establishing charges for the extended care unit; problems would arise in the event a patient was transferred back and forth between units. It is recommended, therefore, that the method used for establishing charges in the acute units and that used for the extended care unit be very similar, if not identical.

It is reasonable to assume that most extended care patients will need occupational and/or recreational therapy. It is wise to consider including these two services in the daily service charge. Justification for this is twofold: greater participation is assured, and the cost is relatively low because extended care patients usually receive these services as a group and not at the same time of day as the acute patients.

Experience indicates that physical therapy, on the other hand, should not be included in the basic rate since to do so encourages inappropriate admission to the unit of patients who should instead be in the intensive rehabilitation unit.

Establishing charges for extended care involves other factors, too. For example, both physicians and patients expect it to be a lower cost unit. The success of the unit in terms of utilization by the physician and the attitude of the patient is based, in part, on this expectation. If charges do not bear this out, it will be difficult to promote utilization of the unit.

Since the major source of financing the operating costs of general hospitals is patient revenue, much of the financing may come from third-party payers. Because the extent of coverage varies not only with the insuring organization, but with the locality, it would be wise to consult with the local Blue Cross Plan and with commercial insurance companies to determine whether their policies include provisions for extended care.

In the case of welfare patients, most welfare agencies have established a rigid payment plan for nursing home care. Because extended care is a fairly new concept, it is conceivable that no payment plan has been established as yet. In this event, it might be wise to point out to the welfare agency that the extended care unit is a unit of a general hospital and, logically, reimbursement should be made on the same basis as for other units of the hospital.

Chapter 4

OPERATING THE EXTENDED CARE UNIT

Generally speaking, the extended care unit would function within the framework of overall hospital policies and procedures. Deviations from general policies or special policies and procedures applicable only to the unit are those made necessary by the unit's divergent objectives.

After policies have been developed and approved, and implementing procedures have been devised, it is recommended that a written statement of these policies be circulated among hospital staff and other appropriate persons. A periodic review of extended care policies will help avoid makeshift accommodation to immediate pressures or decisions made by default.

Ongoing policy formulation then becomes a joint responsibility of the governing board, the administration, the medical director and/or medical staff committee, and the nursing supervisor. Special staff policies applying only to the extended care unit should be incorporated in the hospital medical staff bylaws, rules, and regulations, and those general policies that also apply to extended care should clearly state that the unit is covered by them.

ORGANIZATIONAL STRUCTURE

The organizational structure of the extended care unit should, of course, fit smoothly into the overall hospital structure and be an active part of the ongoing operation. The unit should be organized to permit speed of action and to provide efficient and effective channels of communication.

Responsibility for administrative and clinical direction and for nursing services should be in the hands of people who command authority and respect; responsibility should not be delegated too far downward, however, or given to someone who does not have authority to make decisions.

ADMINISTRATIVE RESPONSIBILITIES

Administrative responsibilities should be delegated to someone who is able to make decisions, interpret policy, and establish the identity of the extended care unit. These responsibilities are particularly important to the overall functioning of the unit.

Making decisions. The person who handles the day-to-day operation of the unit should be one who knows the staff and has daily contact with them—one who can either make decisions or obtain decisions with minimum delay.

Interpreting policy. Particularly in the initial period, special policies adopted for the unit will have to be flexibly interpreted in many specific situations; unexpected problems may require the development of new policies. The person in charge of the unit must have knowledge and understanding of the operation of both the hospital itself and the extended care unit, to ensure that procedures are streamlined and efficient and that general rules are not being rigidly applied when an individual approach is more appropriate.

Establishing identity. To promote understanding of the purpose and function of the unit and to emphasize the advantages of its existence within the hospital complex, there must be a continuing flow of information to the professional staff of the hospital, to the broader medical community, to other health facilities, and to the public. The person who handles this responsibility must have the ability to work with the medical staff, with community leaders, and with the news media.

CLINICAL DIRECTION

It is important that clinical direction of the extended care program be an ongoing responsibility of the medical staff. This may be achieved through appointment of a chief of service—with or without a medical advisory committee—or through the establishment of a medical staff committee responsible for clinical direction and policy determination. If the latter method is chosen, it is essential that the committee authorize one of its members—perhaps the chairman—to act on day-to-day matters.

It is recommended that provisions adopted for the clinical direction of the extended care unit be incorporated into the medical staff bylaws and that specific duties and powers of the chief of service, or of the committee, be agreed upon and put into writing. This provides an excellent basis for formal hospital communication with the medical staff.

Chief of clinical service. The duties of the chief of clinical service (which would apply equally to a committee) have been summarized as follows: *

- To supervise, measure, and evaluate the professional care in the service, being mindful always of the spiritual, physical, psychological, and economic needs of the patient; to strive to maintain adequate, clear, and precise communications with all segments of the hospital complex.
- To plan continually for the growth and upgrading of the service.
- To be concerned with the establishment of a scholarly attitude, using all teaching implementation necessary to carry out a program for education.
- To encourage research, both basic and clinical.
- To have an intimate knowledge of the attending staff; to encourage staff members to abide by the bylaws and to accept their responsibilities of self-education, self-evaluation, and self-criticism.

In essence, extended care is a program of enablement. It is the job of the chief of service—or, in some hospitals, the medical director

*Bizzozero, O. Duties of the clinical service chief. *Hosp. Progr.* 46:81, Jan. 1965.

—to enable the practicing physician to provide comprehensive care, to push for the necessary personnel and the necessary services in the unit, and to promote efficient utilization of the unit through education and active case finding.

Responsibilities of the chief of service are not confined solely to the unit, or even to the hospital. Planning with the attending physician for the continuing care of patients after discharge is also his concern. At the least, this requires effective liaison with other facilities and services and a procedure for transmitting information about the patient when he is transferred; at the most, if outlets are unacceptable or nonexistent, it requires an effort to upgrade existing services or to initiate new ones, such as a teaching program for nursing home personnel in the area, a home care program, or consultation services.

Advisory committee. Representation on a directing or advisory committee will vary with the purpose and programs of the unit. In most instances, however, a broad range of specialties will be involved with the extended care patients, and committee representation should reflect this involvement.

NURSING SERVICES

To ensure prompt action when problems arise and to facilitate efficient functioning, the nursing supervisor of the extended care unit will need to have direct lines of communication with the administration and the chief of service. In this kind of organizational pattern, the nursing, clinical, and administrative leadership of the unit becomes a coordinated management team.

It is important that adequate authority be delegated to the nursing supervisor to permit the development of a nursing staff that is oriented to the objectives of patient care in the extended care unit. She should be free, for example, to assign functions in accordance with nursing needs and the skills of her staff and to recommend policies to meet special requirements of the unit. Although nursing policies should be consistent for the entire hospital, procedures can be adapted to meet the differing needs of extended care patients.

Undoubtedly there are many workable plans of organization for an extended care unit. In choosing one it is well to keep in mind, however, that the initial phases of the operation are particularly important, as is the need for the unit to start off on an equal footing with already established units in the hospital. If, in the beginning, the extended care unit is considered less important than the others, this attitude will be hard to change.

ADMINISTRATIVE PROCEDURES

Administrative procedures in the extended care unit should be patterned after those used in other departments and nursing units, with one addition—the individual patient progress review. This procedure is usually initiated by the nursing supervisor of the unit. In some programs it is done on a weekly basis. Participants generally are the attending or resident physician, the nursing supervisor, the social worker, and the rehabilitation therapist who are actively involved with the patient.

GENERAL MEDICAL STAFF RESPONSIBILITIES

The medical staff's responsibility for patients is the same in the extended care unit as in other units of the hospital, though there might be some difference in the policies concerning frequency of visits and frequency of progress notes.

Other medical staff responsibilities may be carried out through standing committees of the medical staff whose functions should be expanded to cover the extended care unit. These committee functions include pharmacy, tissue, medical records, infection control, and overall appraisal of the quality of medical care, including utilization review.

If it has been decided to permit physicians who are not on the hospital staff to admit patients to this unit only, specific rules and regulations concerning these admissions must be developed. It would be necessary, for example, to have a policy governing the situation in which the patient requires admission to a general hospital. Such a policy would have to delineate the physician's responsibility to accomplish a prompt transfer to another hospital or to arrange with a member of the staff to take responsibility for the patient if the patient is transferred to the acute section of the same hospital.

UTILIZATION REVIEW

Utilization review is designed to ensure prompt and appropriate placement of patients in the total facility, both on admission and during the various phases of their illness; to assess appropriate utilization of facilities and services throughout the patient's stay; to determine the necessity for continuing stay; and to assess the plans developed in advance for the continuing care of patients at home or in other health care facilities.*

The broad concept of regular medical review of patients, to ensure that medical care given to them is both adequate and necessary, is not new. Over the years, activity to improve hospital standards and quality of care has led to the establishment of clinical-pathological conferences, regular medical staff meetings, tissue committees, medical audits, medical record committees, and so on. In long-term care facilities, such as tuberculosis hospitals, periodic staff review of treatment and progress of individual patients—sometimes called staffing or case conferencing—has been routine for years.

The review function for an extended care unit might well be combined with the overall medical care appraisal responsibility. If the hospital does not have a medical staff committee that performs these functions, or if its committee is not functioning effectively, steps should be taken to ensure an efficient review program. Not only is this good medical practice, but it is required by the Joint Commission on Accreditation of Hospitals and by third-party payers, including the federal government through its Medicare program.

The medical staffs of hospitals that provide a wide range of organized health care services are finding it increasingly necessary to develop procedures for reviewing patients' needs in relation to their placement in the appropriate unit. Experimentation is under way in the use of various kinds of health care personnel to relieve the physician of unnecessary time-consuming activities in accomplishing this review, and this should lead to more efficient and economical procedures. For example, a nurse or social worker might assist the attending physician and the medical staff committee by carrying out a quick regular review of patient placement, using criteria developed by the committee. This would reduce the number of decisions that would have to be made by the medical staff committee, which could then review the problem cases, along with a random sample of patients' records, at its regularly scheduled staff meeting. Such a

*American Hospital Association. *Guiding Principles for Utilization Review Programs for Extended Care Facilities.* Chicago: AHA, 1966.

procedure would also ensure the continuing effectiveness of the patient placement program.

Because the extended care unit operates in that part of the spectrum of care between the acute hospital and the skilled nursing home, its success in maintaining that position rests largely on the observance of effective admission and discharge policies and on regular review of performance in relation to them.

MEDICAL AND ADMINISTRATIVE RECORDS

The advantages of using the same medical record forms in all units of the hospital seem to outweigh any gains that might accrue from using forms with minor changes for the extended care unit. With the possible exception of consolidated forms for recording medications, there does not appear to be any significant need for deviation from the standard.

The patient's medical record should accompany him when he is transferred to the extended care unit from another service within the hospital, or vice versa, just as it does when a transfer occurs between the medical and surgical services, for example. It is also customary for a transfer note to be added in which the patient's condition is summarized. Such a summary would include the patient's treatment plan, supported by the necessary orders.

Administrative records need not differ a great deal from records maintained on any other group of patients. This unit, like any other nursing unit, will have its complement of records regarding patients and patient statistics. It is suggested, however, that statistics for this unit be kept separate from those for other units of the hospital for purposes of reporting and of evaluation. This provides an easy means of comparing this unit with others in terms of the use of ancillary services, cost factors, income, service rendered, and other areas critical to the evaluation process. To make the comparisons valid it is wise to maintain a uniform system of reporting; cost finding procedures are desirable because they provide the mechanism for separating the costs of the extended care unit from those of other units.

AMOUNT AND TYPES OF SERVICES

While certain limitations on the amount and types of services offered in the extended care unit merit careful thought, it should be generally understood that the medical and diagnostic services of the hospital are available to any patient who requires them. This includes laboratory, x-ray, pharmacy, electrocardiography, electroencephalography, and so on, as well as the basic rehabilitative services essential to accomplishment of the unit's objectives. Experience indicates, however, that if an extended care patient requires surgery or if his condition becomes such that he is likely to need intensive nursing care for more than a short time, he should be transferred to the acute section.

Limitation of services such as oxygen therapy, intravenous therapy, and blood transfusions is recommended because they require professional supervision by registered nurses, who are usually relatively fewer on the typical extended care unit. Providing these services, except on an infrequent or emergency basis, would mean either that the unit would have to employ a higher ratio of registered nurses (canceling out one factor that may permit a lower daily charge) or that the time of those on the staff would be disproportionately devoted to these problems.

Because the patients admitted to the extended care unit are not expected to show significant changes in their condition as frequently as acutely ill patients, the frequency of certain routine nursing procedures—for example, the measurement of blood pressure, temperature, pulse, and respiration—is subject to specific exceptions on the physician's orders.

It is necessary, of course, to have a report on the condition of patients to transmit at the change of nursing shifts; such reports can be limited, however, to those patients in whom a significant change has occurred or for whom special nursing orders have been written. In brief, both nursing procedures and the recording of information should be geared to the patients served; only those that are meaningful and necessary to their needs for care should be required.*

Dietary service might well be limited to the provision of one special diet in each category of need. Many patient services rendered routinely in the acute hospital—such as the provision of drinking water in every room—can be eliminated in the extended care unit, particularly for patients who are ambulatory and relatively self-sufficient. All patients should be given every opportunity to do things for themselves in preparation for discharge.

*For further information see *Medical Record Departments in Hospitals: Guide to Organization.* Chicago: American Hospital Association, 1972.

STAFF SELECTION AND TRAINING

SELECTION

Selection of the right kind of person as *nursing supervisor* of the unit is particularly important.* The nursing supervisor should be well grounded in rehabilitation nursing, be aware of the psychosocial factors influencing illness and recovery, be able to indoctrinate the staff with rehabilitation concepts and attitudes, and be capable of organizing and directing a continuing inservice education program. If such a person is not available from the hospital staff or other sources, the hospital may select a nurse who has the necessary interest and qualifications and then underwrite whatever additional education or training is required. This additional education or training should be completed before the unit is scheduled to open.

The selection of the *nurse rehabilitation coordinator* is also an important one. The rehabilitation coordinator helps patients to become as proficient as possible in the several activities of daily living, and should also aid the nursing supervisor by providing liaison between nursing and the rehabilitation therapies, by coordinating the restorative efforts within and outside of the unit, and by interpreting to other nursing personnel the relation of rehabilitation objectives to the nursing care program of each patient.

Selection of the nonprofessional staff is actually more difficult than selection of professional nurses. There are requirements for the education and licensure of practical nurses, but there are no standards for the education, training, and experience of aides and orderlies, although their continuing contact with patients makes their role vital. Patience, tact, and understanding are traits every staff member should have, but these traits are not easy to identify. To avoid misconceptions on the part of applicants and to help the interviewer gauge their attitude toward the kinds of patients they would be serving, applicants should always be given a clear picture of the function and purpose of the unit; job descriptions should be reviewed with them; job satisfactions derived from the opportunity to render more individualized service should be pointed out.

TRAINING

Inservice training not only improves patient care by increasing staff competence, but also reduces costs by minimizing staff turn-

*For further information see *Guidelines for the Practice of Nursing on the Rehabilitation Team*. New York: American Nurses' Association, 1965.

over. A strong and continuous inservice program of education and training is particularly important in the extended care unit, because of the high ratio of nonprofessional to professional personnel. The program should cover such subjects as:

1. The extended care unit—its purpose, function, policies and procedures, and the types of patients admitted, as well as its relationship to the hospital as a whole.
2. Activities of daily living, and related staff responsibilities.
3. Rehabilitation nursing—its rationale and fundamental importance.
4. Emotional and social problems of patients and their families; the roles of the social worker and the psychologist.
5. Rehabilitation therapies—their applications to extended care patients, and related staff responsibilities.
6. Mechanics of body movements and lifting (lectures, movies, and demonstrations and return demonstrations by unit personnel).
7. Medical emergencies (movies, lectures, demonstrations and return demonstrations of such measures as resuscitation and external cardiac massage).
8. Team conferences—use of the nursing team concept in preparing plans of care and progress reports on all patients.
9. Staff meetings—general meetings and separate meetings for each category of personnel.

USE OF VOLUNTEERS

Volunteers can become important members of the therapeutic team in an extended care unit. By helping to fill the patients' social and emotional needs, they contribute to higher morale of both the staff and the patients. For the long-term patient, who often feels cut off from the community, the volunteer serves as an important link with the outside world, helping to maintain the patient's identity as an individual and to lessen his preoccupation with his disease or impairment.

Volunteers serving in an extended care unit should have, in addition to the regular volunteer orientation, special training on such subjects as types of chronic illness, general personality characteristics of the long-term patient, and the volunteer's role on the therapeutic team. Volunteers should be included in team training sessions whenever possible.

Although volunteers in extended care units can be used in groups for occupational therapy and recreational activities, they often are assigned on a one-to-one basis. When this is the practice, it is important that the person in charge of volunteers have sufficient information about both the volunteer and the patient to make a suitable assignment. Before each visit the volunteer should be apprised of the patient's condition. How much specific information he receives should be left to the discretion of the medical staff; however, he should at least know the patient's limitations and mental attitude. The volunteer should, of course, report to the supervisor anything unusual that occurs during his visit.

RELATIONSHIP TO EDUCATIONAL PROGRAM

Chronic diseases pose unique problems for the physician and for others. Traditionally the physician has been trained to make a diagnosis and to prescribe the appropriate immediate treatment. In chronic disease there may be no specific treatment for the disease itself; but there may be long-term medical needs relating to factors such as the patient's adaptation pattern, resistance, physical conditioning, use of residual assets, and purpose or goal. These factors call for reevaluation if the long-term patient is to be kept in the mainstream of medical care, a task involving not only the physician, but also other trained personnel, and community resources outside the hospital as well.

In order to provide learning experiences for the physician and for other personnel, every effort should be made to take advantage of the educational opportunities offered by the extended care unit. All health professionals—physicians, residents, interns, medical students, nurses, social workers, and therapists—can benefit from experience with the diversity of patients and illnesses encountered in an extended care unit. Such experience can develop understanding of the importance of rehabilitation nursing, insight into the social and psychological problems of the disabled and the chronically ill, and awareness of the need for early and comprehensive planning for discharge.

One educational approach, for example, might be to have medical students, interns, and residents indicate the prognosis for each patient. Essentially, this prognosis should consider not only the usual natural history of the disease, but also the degree to which the patient is functioning or will function to the limit of his capabilities, and the types of medical facilities and services that he will need over the course of his illness. Will he be readmitted for short periods or longer ones? Will he be transferred to another facility or will he require outpatient care or home care?

PROVISION FOR CONTINUING CARE

If the hospital has an effective program for medical care appraisal and utilization review, it would be reasonable to expect that appropriate patients are being admitted to the extended care unit and that they are receiving the kind of care they require. Further, it could be expected that patients are being recommended for discharge when measurable and significant gains can no longer be observed.

Of equal importance, however, is the mechanism the hospital sets up to provide for the patient's continuing care—whether that care be given in his home or in another health care facility such as a nursing home.

Working agreements between the hospital and outside resources of assured quality are recommended. These agreements, like policies concerning the transfer of hospital patients to and from the unit, should be reciprocal. Patients and their families are more likely to accept a move if they can be reasonably sure that the patient will be readmitted to the original facility, should that become necessary.

In a community where a sufficient range of alternative programs is not available, the general hospital has the responsibility for encouraging the development of such programs or increasing the scope of its own services. Often the general hospital is the center of the community's medical resources; it has, therefore, the organizational experience on which to build a coordinated system of patient care, and it also has the necessary foundation of community respect and confidence.

While outlets for discharge are essential, their availability does not in itself guarantee a genuine continuum of high-quality care. Planning for transfer, and particularly for discharge, requires social as well as medical evaluation; casework help is invaluable in making suitable discharge arrangements and in carrying them out.

Not only is it important that patient care be uninterrupted, but it is equally important that the patient experience a sense of "wholeness" in his plan of care. Too often, a patient transferred from one unit to another or from one facility to another does not perceive, and is not helped to understand, that these moves are being made in his own best interest. This makes adjustment to the new situation difficult for both patient and staff, and may seriously affect the patient's welfare. One way to help the patient adjust is to encourage visits to him, while he is still in the hospital, by personnel from the agency or facility to which the patient is being transferred. Thus, when the patient arrives in the new, strange place, or is visited at home, he will see at least one familiar face.

The transmittal of information about the patient's condition and his continuing care needs is also vitally important. Carefully constructed referral forms are useful (see form on next two pages). A review of the patient's record by a staff member from the facility the patient is entering, or by the public health nurse, or by a counselor from a public agency should help in providing a continuum of high-quality care. If the patient is going home, it is important that his family be given clear instructions—both oral and written—concerning the care he will require.

RELATIONSHIPS OUTSIDE THE HOSPITAL

Once people understand what is meant by extended care and how the patient can benefit from it, they are usually more willing to support it. To promote this understanding, all techniques for community education should be utilized. Continuing education of the medical staff, and through them, education of the broader medical community, is basic. Other approaches worth exploring are orientation programs for health insurance representatives, for attorneys and trust officers of banks, and for secretaries and nurses in physicians' offices.

REVIEW AND EVALUATION OF PROGRAM

A mechanism should be established for a periodic review of the entire extended care program to compare its performance with stated therapeutic and social goals. The medical staff committee directing or advising the unit should review, together with the administration, the clinical operational policies, as well as the overall goals of the program. Nursing services should also be

PATIENT TRANSFER FORM

Name ____________ (LAST) ____________ (FIRST) ____________

Age ______ Sex ______ Religion ____________ Soc. Sec. # ____________

Relative or Guardian ____________ (RELATION)

Relative or Guardian's Address ____________ Tel. ____________

From ____________ Admission ____________

Address ____________

Date of Transfer ____________

Transferred to ____________ (HOSP., NURSING HOME, AGENCY)

Address ____________

Clinic Appt. ____________

Date and Time ____________

____________ (ATTACH CLINIC APPOINTMENT CARD)

Physician in Charge at Time of Transfer ____________ M.D.

Will this Physician care for Patient after Admission to Nursing Home? ______

II. MAJOR DIAGNOSES

(Check if present)

Disabilities
- Amputation
- Paralysis
- Contracture
- Decub. Ulcer

Impairments
- Mentality
- Speech
- Hearing
- Vision
- Sensation

Incontinence
- Bladder
- Bowel
- Saliva

Activity Tolerance Limitations
- None
- Moderate
- Severe

Patient knows diagnosis?

IMPORTANT MEDICAL INFORMATION

(State allergies if any)

DIET, DRUGS, AND OTHER THERAPY

at Time of Discharge

(Physician, please sign below)

Chest X-ray	date ______	result ______
C.B.C.	date ______	result ______
Serology	date ______	result ______
Urinalysis	date ______	result ______

SUGGESTIONS FOR ACTIVE CARE

BED

Position in good body alignment and change position every ______ hrs.

Avoid ____________ position

Prone position ______ times/day as tolerated.

SIT IN CHAIR

______ hrs. ______ times/day.

WEIGHT BEARING

Full ______ Partial ______ None ______

on ____________ leg

LOCOMOTION

Walk ____________ times/day.

EXERCISES

Range of motion ____________ times/day

to ____________

by patient ______ nurse ______ family ______.

Other as outlined below ____________.

Stand ______ Min. ______ times/day.

SOCIAL ACTIVITIES

Encourage group ______ individual ______

within ______ outside ______ home.

Transport: Ambulance ______ Car ______

Car for handicapped ______ Bus ______

SUGGESTIONS FOR COMPLETING FORM

1. The purpose of this form is to insure continuity of care in transfer from hospital to home or home to hospital.
2. The form is not intended to supply information of long-term nature.
3. Original should accompany patient with transfer. Carbon retained in patient's record.

Signature of Physician or Nurse ____________ Date ____________

Patient transfer form, page 1. (See next page for page 2.)

Prepared by the Chicago Hospital Council and the Chicago Nursing Home Association.

III. PATIENT INFORMATION

SELF CARE STATUS

(Check level of ability. Write S in space if needs supervision only. Draw line across if inapplicable.)

	Independent	Needs Assistance	Unable to do	
Bed Activity				Turns
				Sits
Personal Hygiene				Face, Hair, Arms
				Trunk & Perineum
				Lower Extremities
				Bladder Program
				Bowel Program
Dressing				Upper Extremities
				Trunk
				Lower Extremities
				Appliance, Splint
				Feeding
Transfer				Sitting
				Standing
				Tub
				Toilet
Locomotion				Wheelchair
				Walking
				Stairs

BED Low____ Mattress: Firm____ Reg.____
Other____
Side Rails: Yes____ No____

BEHAVIOR
Alcoholic____ Belligerent____ Noisy____
Senile____ Suspicious____ Withdrawn____

MENTAL STATUS
Alert____ Forgetful____ Confused____

COMMUNICATION ABILITY	Yes	No
Can speak		
Can write		
Understands speaking		
Understands writing		
Understands gestures		
Understands English		

If no, state language spoken:____

DIET
Regular____ Low Salt____ Diabetic____
Bland____ Low Residue____
Feeds self____ Needs help____
Part____ All____

PATIENT USES
Appliance____ Catheter____ Colostomy____
Cane____ Crutches____ Prosthesis____
Walker____ Chair____

OTHER EQUIPMENT ____

ADDITIONAL PERTINENT INFORMATION

(Explain necessary details of care, diagnosis, medications, treatments, prognosis, teaching, habits, preferences, etc. Therapists and social workers add signature and title to notes.)

IV. SOCIAL INFORMATION

(Adjustment to disability, emotional support from family, motivation for self care, socializing ability, financial plan, family health problem, etc.)

Social Welfare Agencies Active____ Signature____ Title:____ Date:____

Patient transfer form, page 2.

evaluated.* Other departments of the hospital—particularly physical therapy, occupational therapy, and social service—should periodically analyze the amount and efficacy of their work with extended care patients; such an analysis would include: number of patients seen; number and type of treatments or service given; increases or decreases, and the reasons therefor; and an evaluation of the results. The actual use of ancillary services should also be compared with their expected use. The reasons for such a comparison are: (1) to assess the impact of the extended care unit and (2) to determine through utilization whether patient selection has been appropriate.

Answers to certain key questions in a number of areas will help in evaluating the total extended care program. Some of these questions are as follows.

OBJECTIVES

- Are patients in the unit the types for which the service was planned?
- Have objectives changed? If so, were the changes planned? Is everyone concerned aware of the changes?
- What is the ratio of direct admissions to transfers? Is this ratio appropriate in terms of the objectives of the unit?

UTILIZATION

- Does the medical staff understand the unit's function and use the unit appropriately?
- Is the method of charging deterring the use of special services? Are enough services included in the basic rate?

QUALITY OF CARE

- Have nursing care needs increased in scope and in amount? Have there been corresponding adjustments in staffing?
- Are extended care patients getting appropriate physician supervision? If not, do the medical staff rules and regulations need strengthening?

*Veterans Administration, Department of Medicine and Surgery. *Nursing Care of the Long-Term Patient,* Program Guide, Nursing Service #G-8, M-2, Part V. Washington, D.C.: U.S. Government Printing Office, 1963, Chap. 4.

- Is the recreational therapy program appropriate for the kinds of patients accepted?
- Are the social and emotional aspects of extended care receiving sufficient emphasis? Is the social work staffing adequate to meet the patients' needs?

CONTINUING CARE

- Are patients getting the kind of continuing care they need after discharge? If not, is this due to inadequacy of other health care resources in the community, or to a lack of proper arrangements with them?

COSTS AND CHARGES

- Is the unit financially stable?
- How do costs in this unit compare with those of a medical-surgical unit?
- If charges are lower, are costs really lower when the same method of allocating costs is used?
- Are extended care patients being subsidized by other hospital patients?

GENERAL

- How do the patients and their families react to this type of care? If they are dissatisfied, is it because of lack of proper orientation or because the unit is not functioning well?

GENERAL REFERENCES

BOOKS AND MANUALS

PUBLICATIONS OF THE AMERICAN HOSPITAL ASSOCIATION

American Hospital Association. *American Hospital Association Guide to the Health Care Field*. Chicago: AHA, 1972.

———. *Essentials of Social Work Programs in Hospitals*. Chicago: AHA, 1971.

———. *Guiding Principles for Utilization Review Programs for Extended Care Facilities*. Chicago: AHA, 1966.

———. *Hospital Design Checklist*. Chicago: AHA, 1965.

———. *Medical Record Departments in Hospitals: Guide to Organization*. Chicago: AHA, 1972.

———. *Meeting the Social Needs of Long-Term Patients*. Chicago: AHA, 1965.

———. *Physical Therapy Service: A Guide to Organization and Management*. Chicago: AHA, 1965.

———. *Principles of Organization, Management, and Community Relations for Hospitals.* Chicago: AHA, 1964.

———. *Rehabilitation Services in Hospitals and Related Facilities: A Guide to Planning, Organization, and Management.* Chicago: AHA, 1966.

———. *Relationships among Health Care Facilities.* Chicago: AHA, 1965.

———. *Statement on Optimum Health Services.* Chicago: AHA, 1965.

Littauer, D. *et al. A Chronic Disease Unit in a General Hospital: Analysis of Six Years' Operating Experience.* Chicago: American Hospital Association, 1963.

PUBLICATIONS FROM OTHER SOURCES

American Nurses' Association. *Guidelines for the Practice of Nursing on the Rehabilitation Team.* New York: ANA, 1965.

Beamer, D. E. *Operation of a Nursing Home by the General Hospital.* Abstract. Richmond: Medical College of Virginia, 1962.

Commission on Chronic Illness. *Chronic Illness in the United States,* Vol. II, *Care of the Long-Term Patient.* Cambridge, Mass.: Harvard University Press, 1956.

Ferguson, T., and MacPhail, A. N. *Hospital and Community.* London: Oxford University Press, 1954.

Green, W. H. Jr. *Chronic Disease and the Long-Term Unit in the General Hospital.* Richmond: Medical College of Virginia, 1961.

Hospital Review and Planning Council of Southern New York, Inc. *Guide and Suggested Procedures for Use by a Hospital Long-Range Planning and Development Committee.* New York: The Council, 1964.

Joint Committee of the American Hospital Association and the Public Health Service. *Areawide Planning of Facilities for Long-Term Treatment and Care;* report. Washington, D.C.: U.S. Government Printing Office, 1963. (PHS Pub. No. 930-B-1)

Joint Committee of the American Hospital Association and the Public Health Service on Areawide Planning of Hospitals and Related Health Facilities. *Areawide Planning for Hospitals and Related*

Health Facilities; report. Washington, D.C.: U.S. Department of Health, Education, and Welfare, Public Health Service, Division of Hospital and Medical Facilities, 1961. (PHS Pub. No. 855)

Nicholson, E. E. *Planning New Institutional Facilities for Long-Term Care.* New York: G. P. Putnam's Sons, 1956.

Rice, K. D. Organization of long-term care in general hospitals—a comparative study of patterns and practices in a national sample of general hospitals. Unpublished paper, Medical Care Research Center, Washington University, St. Louis, no date.

Salmon, F. C., and Salmon, C. *Rehabilitation Center Planning: An Architectural Guide.* University Park, Pa.: Pennsylvania State University Press, 1959.

U. S. Department of Health, Education, and Welfare, Public Health Service. *General Standards of Construction and Equipment, Long-Term Care Facilities.* Washington, D.C.: U.S. Government Printing Office, 1962.

Veterans Administration, Department of Medicine and Surgery. *Nursing Care of the Long-Term Patient,* Program Guide, Nursing Service #G-8, M-2, Part V. Washington, D.C.: U.S. Government Printing Office, 1963.

ARTICLES

Bizzozero, O. J. Duties of the clinical service chief. *Hosp. Progr.* 46:81, Jan. 1965.

Blair, D. C. Concept of care—treatment. *Can. Hosp.* 39:74, Oct. 1962.

Brown, R. E. General hospital has a general responsibility. *Hospitals, J.A.H.A.* 39:47, June 16, 1965.

Conner, J. F. How we set up our intermediate hospital unit. *Hosp. Manage.* 79:43, May 1955.

Erickson, E. R., and Pedersen, E. Design criteria for a rehabilitation unit. *Hospitals, J.A.H.A.* 39:53, Mar. 1, 1965.

Greco, J. T. Carpeting vs. resilient flooring. *Hospitals, J.A.H.A.* 39:55, June 16, 1965.

Hall, L. E. A center for nursing. *Nurs. Outlook* 11:805, Nov. 1963.

Holland, C. D. How two hospitals met the growing demand for long-term care: Greenville, Ky. *Hospitals, J.A.H.A.* 39:72, June 1, 1965.

Johnson, J. C. Concept of care—convalescent-rehabilitation wing, Calgary General Hospital. *Can. Hosp.* 39:70, Oct. 1962.

Kleh, J. Three roles of the physician in long-term care programs. *Hospitals, J.A.H.A.* 39:63, July 1, 1965.

Marinakos, P. A. Proposal for coordinating hospital and nursing-home services. *Hosp. Top.* 43:33, Apr. 1965.

Novick, L. J. What makes chronic disease hospital administration different? *Hospitals, J.A.H.A.* 38:46, Mar. 16, 1964.

Pick, O. M. How two hospitals met the growing demand for long-term care: Sauk Prairie, Wis. *Hospitals, J.A.H.A.* 39:73, June 1, 1965.

Stevens, D. S. Concept of care—hospital design. *Can. Hosp.* 39:72, Oct. 1962.